POSITIVE VIBES ONLY SYNDROME

21 DAYS OF AFFIRMATIONS FOR PRODUCTIVITY & PEACE

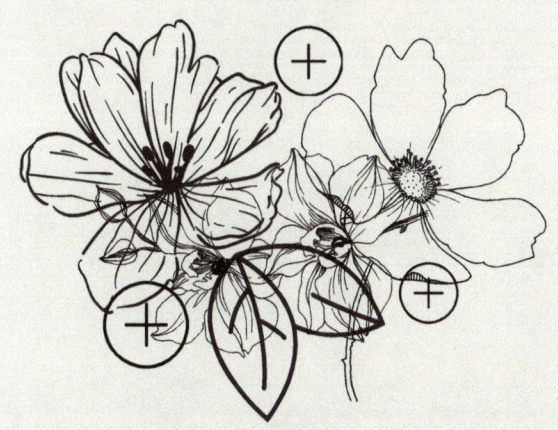

SHONTERAL LAKAY REDMOND, DDS

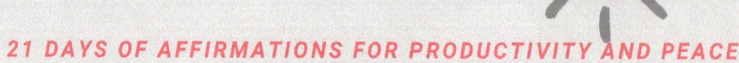

21 DAYS OF AFFIRMATIONS FOR PRODUCTIVITY AND PEACE

POSITIVE VIBES ONLY SYNDROME

1ST EDITION
COPYRIGHT ©2021 BY SHONTERAL LAKAY REDMOND, DDS.
ALL RIGHTS RESERVED.
PUBLISHED BY DR. SHON INC., NEW YORK.
JUNE 21, 2021
DRSHON.COM
ISBN: 978-1-7376045-2-5
DO NOT REPRODUCE WITHOUT WRITTEN PERMISSION.
CONTACT INFO@DRSHON.COM
INSTAGRAM: @DRSHONCOLLEGE | @DRSHONTV | @HOOD2HOODED
TWITTER: @DRSHONTV @DDJSCHOLARS
YOUTUBE: DR. SHON TV | HOOD2HOODED TV | MOTIVATIONAL DENTISTRY TV
TIKTOK: @DRSHONCOLLEGE | @DRSHONTV
IG: @DDJSCHOLARS @DREAMERGENCYWALK

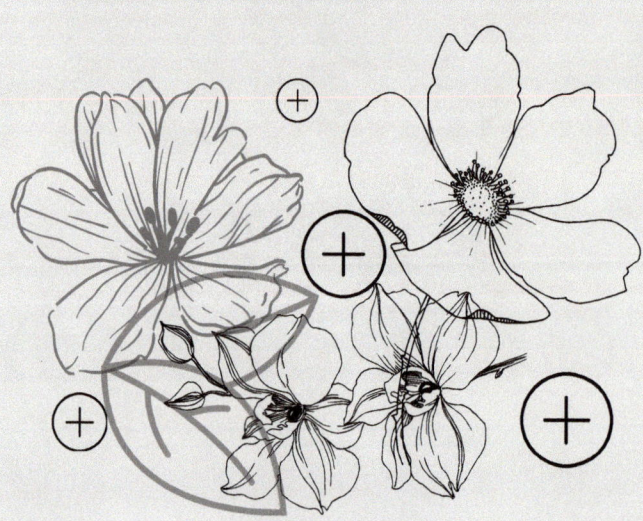

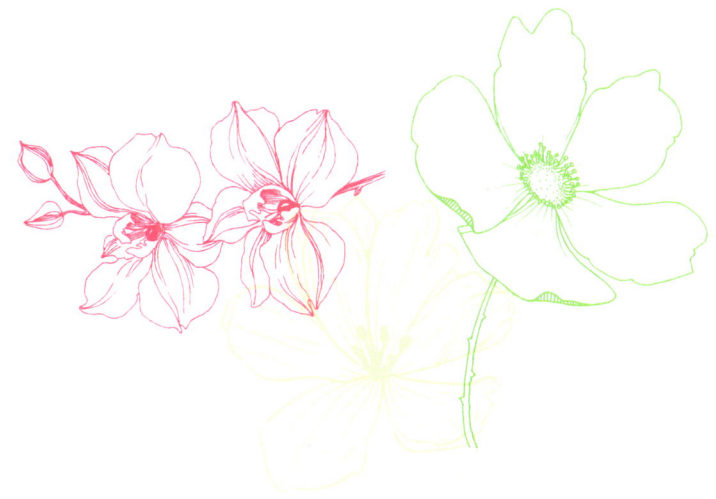

Dedicated to my Mommy in heaven, Doris Denise Jackson,
My Granny, Eartha Lee Gallon,
& the absolute love of my life, Daddy D
(Thank you for always being my #1 inspiration)

-Dr. Shon

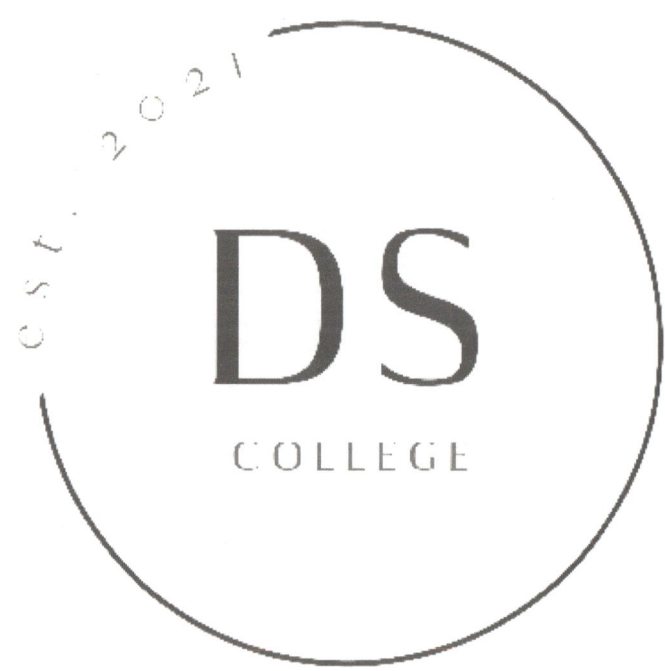

Dr. Shon Inc.

SENDING POSITIVE VIBES ONLY! IT'S A SYNDROME!

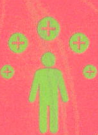

01 INTRODUCTION
DR. SHON THE MOTIVATIONAL DENTIST

08 P.V.O.S. DEFINED
WHAT IS POSITIVE VIBES ONLY SYNDROME?

10 DAILY AFFIRMATIONS
21 DAYS OF PVOS

33 MAINTENANCE
PROPEL INTO THE NEXT LEVEL!
KEEP THOSE POSITIVE VIBES FLOWING!

34 JOURNAL PAGES
DOCUMENT YOUR POSITIVE THOUGHTS

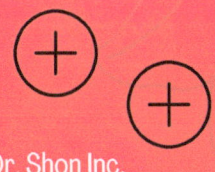

Dr. Shon Inc.

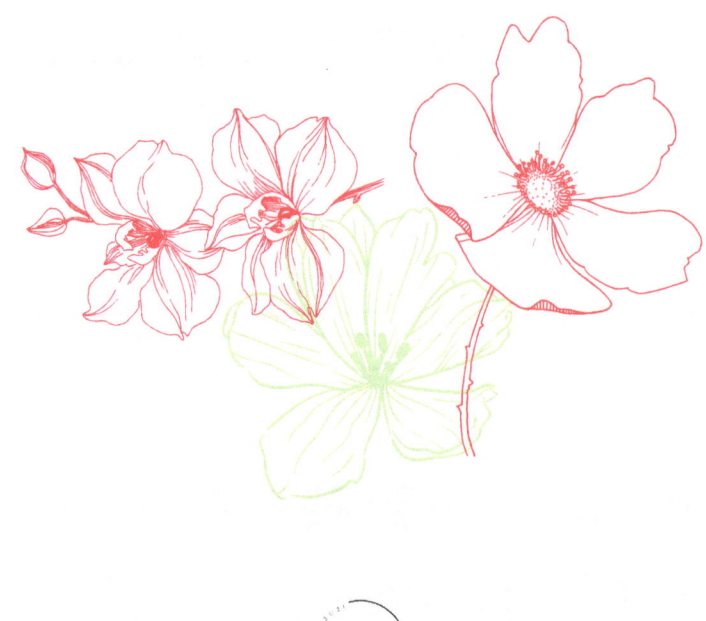

DS

Dr. Shon Inc.

SENDING POSITIVE VIBES ONLY! IT'S A SYNDROME!

Introduction

Writing Positive Vibes Only Syndrome was inspired by a desire to encourage others to live their best life, unapologetically, one day at a time amid the daily stress that threatens our happiness. This book contains short daily readings that promote an uplifting mood and a more inspirational outlook on life. It's designed with a 21-day structure, that as you read, you complete a task daily to build a habit. I believe you can make Positive Vibes Only Syndrome a Habit and a Lifestyle.

If you desire to bring all your wildest dreams to fruition, then you should know that faith is undoubtedly the root of all dreams. "Faith is the assurance of things hoped for, the conviction of things not seen" (Hebrew 11:1). I'm a firm believer in having faith in all one does as it is inevitable. We shouldn't hesitate to embark on a new journey or step out on faith in a new area of life, realizing that God has given us permission to bloom in any area of life we desire.

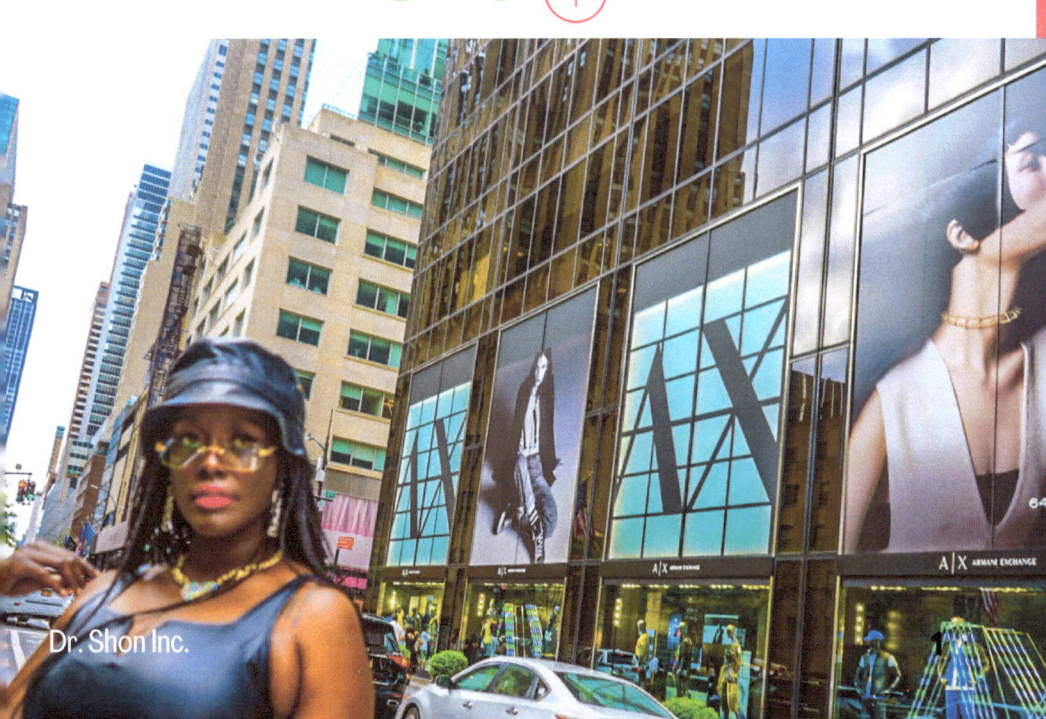

Introduction

    And trust me, you can bloom anytime you desire! To bloom into the best version of yourself, it is imperative that you adjust your mindset to a more positive perspective. This is an unavoidable shift. Through this 21-day experience, steadfast focus and consistency will be crucial to your positive vibes only success! Always remember, despite the turmoil life dishes our way, God is always lifting the heavy load from the path towards our dreams. Spiritual affirmations and self-maintenance are vital to growing stronger.

    Positive Vibes Only Syndrome energy has a way of rebuking mental wounds and scars. We must learn to heal from the inside out. Being unable to escape pain and suffering will always threaten your ability to achieve. Learn to develop a clear ambition and focus of your strengths. Execution of your goals and sacrifice are the master keys to elevation above the odds, as although God makes a way out of no way, you still must do some work. As the times change, pay special attention to the quality of your health, mental clarity, and personal development. These things are essential to continued elevation and growth.

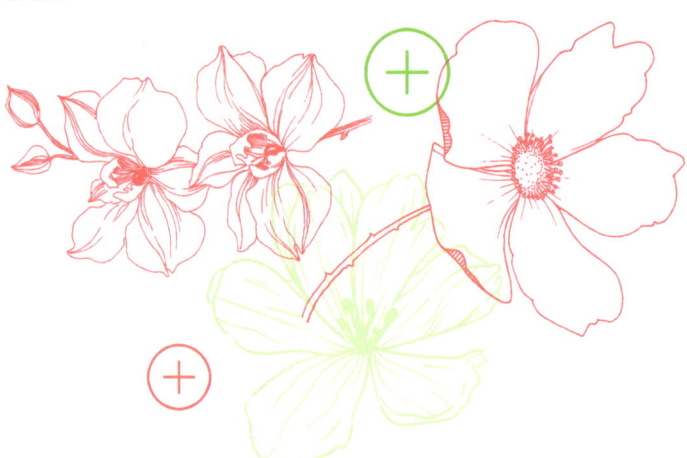

> **POSITIVE VIBES ONLY SYNDROME ENERGY HAS A WAY OF REBUKING MENTAL WOUNDS AND SCARS. WE MUST LEARN TO HEAL FROM THE INSIDE OUT.**

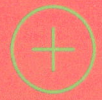
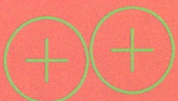

DR. SHON
THE MOTIVATIONAL DENTIST

Introduction

Throughout this e-book, you will find daily affirmations to ignite your positive energy! Use these short phrases to create your own (see sample journal pages) and empower your mind to stay positive at all times.

Stay the course, Kings & Queens; remember, you are not alone.

Cheers to Positive Vibes ONLY Syndrome!

- Shonteral Lakay Redmond, DDS
NYC

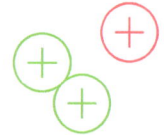

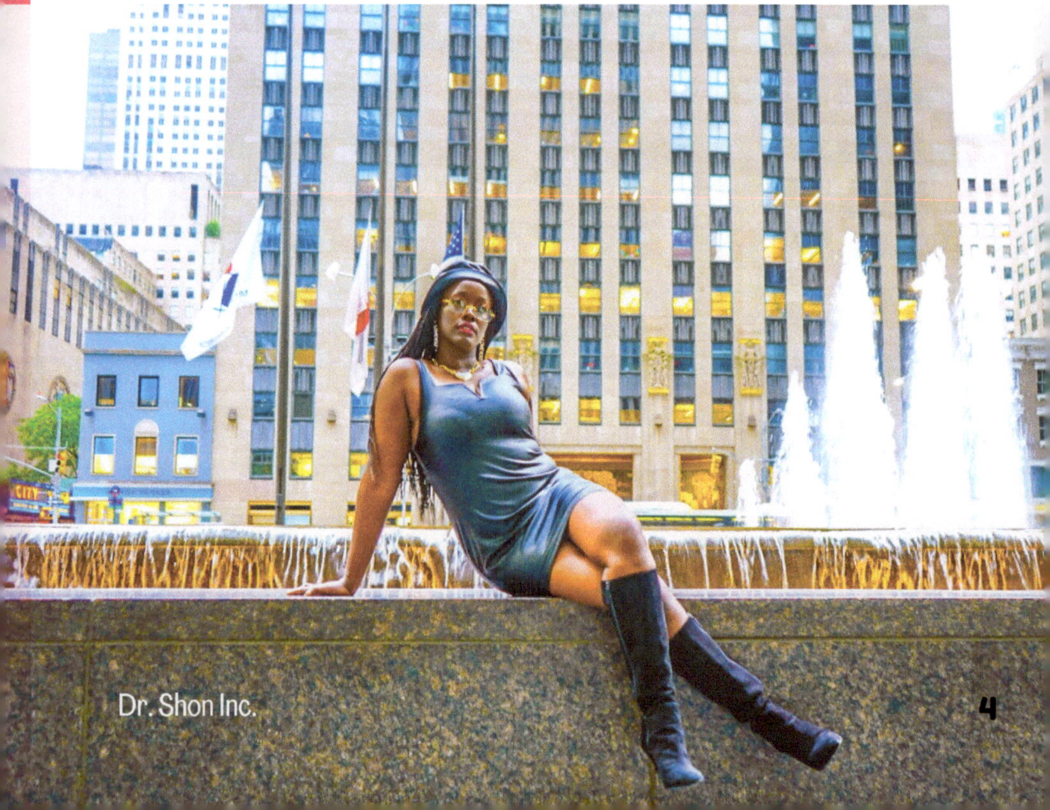

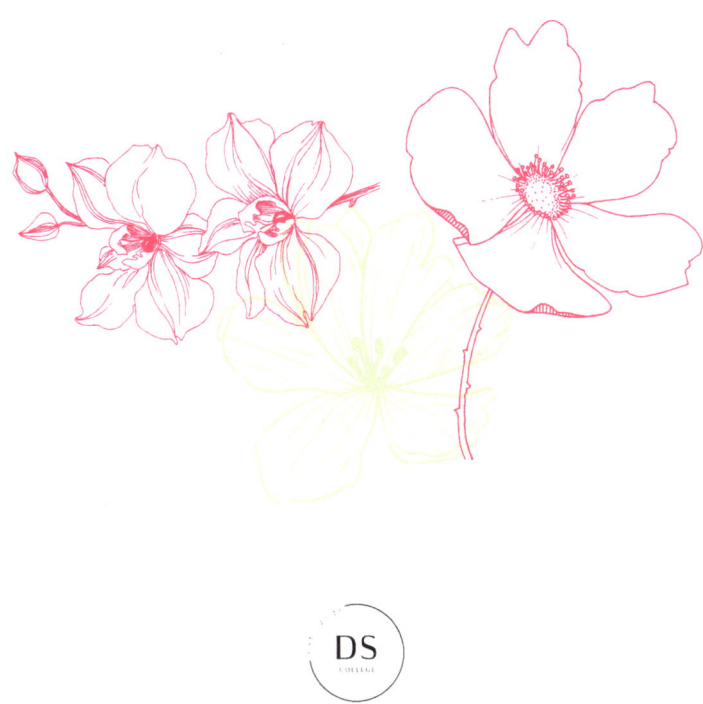

Dr. Shon Inc.

SENDING POSITIVE VIBES ONLY! IT'S A SYNDROME!

Practice Makes Perfect

 **REPEAT THIS AFFIRMATION 3 TIMES**

I WILL WIN BECAUSE I WILL NEVER QUIT ON MYSELF.
I HAVE ENOUGH HOPE AND FAITH TO DRIVE MY DREAMS TO FRUITION.
I WILL MANIFEST ALL THAT I DESIRE FROM THE DEPTHS OF MY SOUL.
GOD IS CONSTANTLY SHOWING OUT AND PROVIDING FOR ALL MY NEEDS.

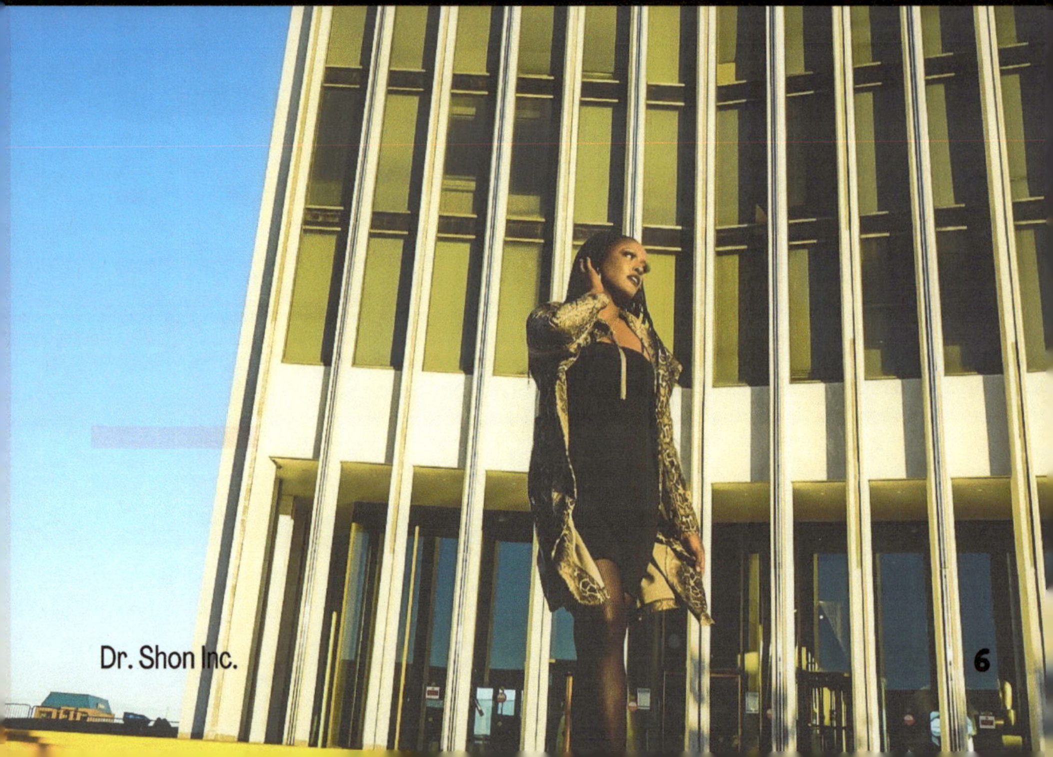

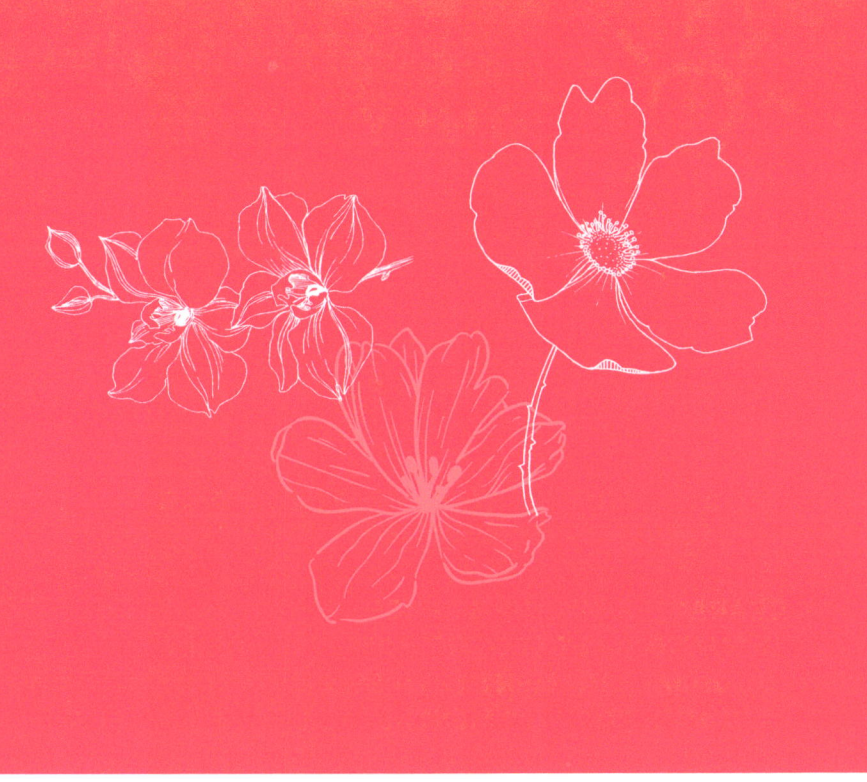

Meditation Moment

Set a timer for 5- 10 minutes.
Find a quiet place to sit alone (DO NOT DISTURB).
Close your eyes. Take slow, intentional deep breaths.
Block out all thoughts that come to your mind.
Envision being surrounded by peace and serenity.
Listen to the responses from your calmer mind.
After the timer ends, journal your thoughts.

Dr. Shon Inc.

SENDING POSITIVE VIBES ONLY! IT'S A SYNDROME!

Positive Vibes ONLY Syndrome DEFINED

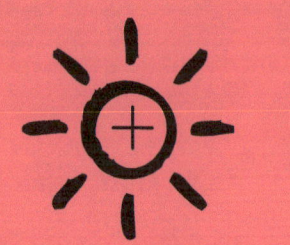
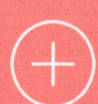

POSITIVE VIBES **ONLY** SYNDROME

PHASE 1
- NEGATIVE ENERGY/ATMOSPHERE SHEDDING

PHASE 2
- CHARACTER BUILDING PHASE
- INTENTIONALLY SEEKING POSITIVITY DAILY
- MOOD MANAGEMENT WITH SELF-TALK
- BUILDING POSITIVE MENTAL BALANCE WITH DAILY AFFIRMATIONS
- NEGATIVITY BLOCKERS — TOOLS THAT DISALLOW THE INTERRUPTION OF POSITIVE ENERGY FLOW

PHASE 3
- MAINTENANCE PHASE
- NEGATIVITY TRIGGER AWARENESS
- PLAN AND PRACTICE MECHANISMS TO AVOID NEGATIVITY, I.E., DEEP BREATHING, WALKING
- PRACTICE/CREATE AFFIRMATIONS CONSISTENTLY
- JOURNAL YOUR POSITIVE EMOTIONS

ARE YOU READY TO TRANSFORM YOUR ENERGY?

Dr. Shon Inc.

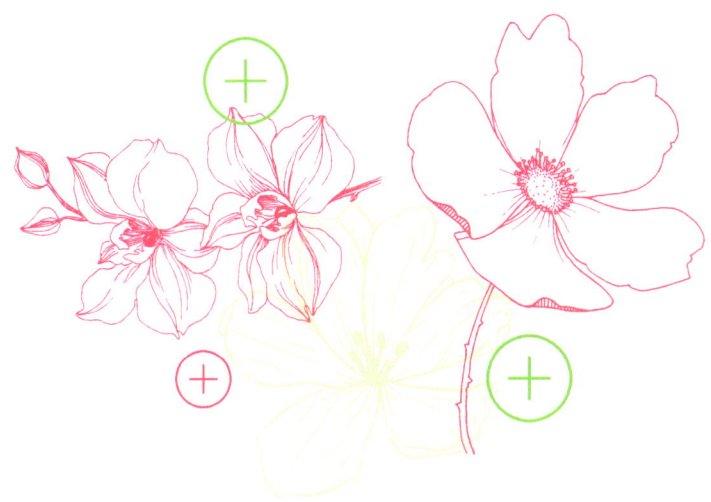

Dr. Shon Inc.

SENDING POSITIVE VIBES ONLY! IT'S A SYNDROME!

DAY 1
I WILL DREAM UP AND NOT DOWN!

In this season, keep your head high and remain focused on your true passions. Never give up on chasing your dreams, or you'll spend your most precious years working for someone else's dream or company. True passions may not pay the bills, initially, but knowledge is free, and knowledge is power. Passions drive you towards your purpose with a greater reward if you stick with it.

Try these positive actions: Pray at least twice today, asking God for your most positive desires with specificity. Ask him for that five-bedroom home on five acres of land or that new job eight times the pay. Ask him to heal a broken heart and give you a renewed strength to open that dream business. Ask for the strength to study for the test you've dreaded so long.

(Continue on next page)

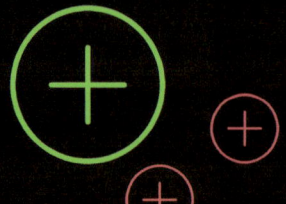

DAY 1
I WILL DREAM UP AND NOT DOWN!

Consider others in your daily efforts of kindness. Be kind to a stranger or even pay it forward. Express self-love, enjoy who you are growing into. Show compassion for yourself and your efforts. Use meditation as a method to gain internal creativity and clarity. Eat organically-grown nutritious foods as often as possible. Bad food only leads to bad vibes.

Simple ethics in life encourage us to cherish our parents, especially if they are still alive. Read daily, as to lead anyone (even yourself), you must be a reader.

Write your goals down every morning. Be a goal digger and generate your own wealth instead of being a gold digger, relying on other folks' wealth.

 Repeat this affirmation 3 times

I will always keep my invisible crown on.
I will only pursue my dreams to phenomenal standards.
I will dream up and never down.

DAY 2
IT'S A FACT THAT THERE ARE MIRACLES IN PROGRESS.

It may feel like we're at a standstill, but God is moving! Press forward with your head held high. You're capable of enduring all your good and bad days with positivity. Please allow God the energy and time to do his miraculous work in your life! Complaining about the hurdles won't make them disappear, instead, learn to pray through the process.

Remember, miraculous things don't happen overnight, so remain patient and faithful. But, with an abundance of positivity and faith, great things will happen overnight, or maybe over the next season of your life. Pretend that your goals and dreams are a garden. Use that energy to find a positive outlook for your situation. Look at the glass as half full. Pessimism will ruin your day, so stay clear of pessimistic people and places. Your energy, aura, and atmosphere should seek to attract nothing but positive vibes—things that make you feel free, happy, energetic, and optimistic about life. Be patient during your growing season, as this is the time to continuously water your garden of goals. Once you've planted the seed, speak positively to your buds until they produce magnificent flowers.

Own your positive vibes only!

 Repeat this affirmation 3 times

Please move in my life, God. I know it is worth the wait! My seeds have been planted, and I believe in myself. I will manifest all my desires through sacrifice, faith, and consistency. I am ready to grow.

Day 3
ALWAYS EXPRESS GRATITUDE

Amid your storm or on your good days, no matter what, give thanks! There is so much to be grateful for. Be grateful for another year of life. Be thankful for your ability to talk, walk and breathe. Be grateful for the good that comes into your life, for all the lessons that appear to test your strength and make you indestructible. Understand and appreciate the lessons learned from the bad news and bad vibes that come your way.

Everything doesn't require your response, as once you respond to negativity, you've been infected with bad vibes. Every day, every moment you feel depressed, down, unclear, unstable, or confused about your energy, pray. Pray for the ability to stay balanced in prayer even during the bad and dark moments. For they are only temporary. Be grateful for the experience you're learning.

This is only a test!

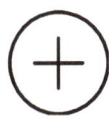

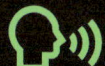
Repeat this affirmation 3 times

DAY 4
EXUDE GREATNESS ON YOUR JOURNEY. ⊕

Now is the time to accept no less than greatness from yourself. Remove the fear that keeps you from detaching from anything less than greatness. You deserve the best. You deserve to feel your best and greatest self daily. Make loving yourself a life's mission. There is no time to feel down or sad about who you are. You were born great. Disallow yourself to continue blaming others for your failures. Everything that you are depends on what decisions and goals you set from this moment forward. Will you rise despite your past? Will you exude greatness in every level of your being?

Don't waste your life allowing folks to treat you in ways you do not want. Disallow your mind to absorb nonsense or useless information that fails to properly heal your mind. Accepting negativity or being in a nonproductive environment will perpetuate the generations of curses preventing you from achieving your highest aspirations. Exercise your free right to access and appreciate knowledge because it is the key to success and happiness. Knowledge can be in any subject or format. Advocate for the advancement of the mind.

 Repeat this affirmation 3 times

I will transform my life into one that seeks knowledge instead of avoiding it.
I will pick up a book and learn new skills that will help me overcome any obstacle I may face.
I have a blessed life.

DAY 5
GOD STILL ANSWERS PRAYERS!

Even when we fail to recognize the blessing inside the test, God will still reveal the magnitude of prayer. The things we desire, write down on paper and speak into existence will one day manifest. And soon too. Everyone wants things to be perfect, but the truth is, we all sometimes fall (most people are just too prideful to be that honest). God still qualifies our voice to inspire others even when we feel unworthy. During the night, pray for the strength to break free from the fear of failing. Pray for a renewed sense of hope.

The beauty in life lies in appreciating the ability to recognize your weakness and get back up again and again.

Repeat this affirmation 3 times

What God has for me is for me, and NO ONE can take that away.
I'm going to break the generational curse no matter how long it may take.
I'm going to live within my purpose and be free, no matter who attempts to get in the way. They will not win. God has me covered!

Dr. Shon Inc.

DAY 6
STORMS DON'T LAST FOREVER.

God prepared us with an innate mental umbrella to help us weather any difficulty that enters our life. It doesn't matter if this is a snowstorm, thunderstorm, hurricane, tornado or straight Blizzard. You have everything inside of you to withstand it and come out on the other side one hundred times better than before. If you get knocked down nine times, then you must get up ten times. If you get knocked down nineteen times, then you must get up twenty times. If you get knocked down one hundred times, you must get up one hundred + one times.

So basically, no matter what happens, always rise back up, always. These storms, rain and season changes should not be an excuse for you to quit. This isn't an excuse for you to just throw in the towel. Just know that your season is coming up again. We all go through ups and lows that make us feel as if life is moving backward, but the further you go back, the further you can go forward. So don't look at these tough times as the end. This is just the beginning.

Positive Vibes ONLY Syndrome is a marathon, NOT a sprint.

⊕

Repeat this affirmation 3 times

I will survive the storm. I am ready to walk into my season unapologetically and fearlessly.

DAY 7
POSITIVITY DOESN'T MIX WITH NEGATIVITY!

If you notice folk fleeing from your good vibes, be thankful. Refuse to allow negative folk to take up your space. Make more room for your blessing! It's time to do some soul cleaning!

Remember, other people can't bless you like God can bless you! To receive the level of respect we desire... We must first initiate that level of respect to others without any expectations of receiving it back. Other folks' standards should never dictate our standards because we don't know who raised them! But as Kings & Queens, we are the example of our creators' love; we show them how it's done. Increase our standards. Increase our blessings. We will exceed all our expectations. There are new blessings headed our way!

 Repeat this affirmation 3 times

I woke up today to be great! Something wonderful is going to happen to me today! Every day God wakes us, we are winning

DAY 8
EXCEPTIONAL FORTITUDE DEFAMES THE STRUGGLES OF THE HOOD'S REALITIES.

    Now is the time to reject defeat and focus on our dreams, goals, and future every day. Learn to express the passion you need to push through tough times. Today, be thankful for all that creates our sense of spiritual being. Worry less about things and people that force you to detach from your spiritual coat. Focus on that which builds your spiritual coat—prayer. No matter who stays by your side or abandons the pride.

    God is always there, and for this reason, be satisfied. Keep your day to life moving on a positive note. When idiots come to ruin the day, don't even give them pleasure in having that opportunity. Talk to God and ask him for cover and shielding against negative spirits. He will comfort your soul and make you impermeable to infected negative folks.

    God is always eager to hear from us! Crowns On.

Repeat this affirmation 3 times

I am in full control of my energy.
I will not allow idiots to ruin my day.
I will approach the day with prayer!

DAY 9
YOU CAN BE AS DOPE AS YOU WANT WITH A LITTLE BIT OF FAITH.

If you're too afraid to live your true purpose, God just may give it to someone who desires it more! Kings & Queens, it's time to unapologetically dance into your favorable destiny. Don't expect success if you aren't willing to do the work. In some lanes, even money can't make you happy with where you are in life. In this situation, you must learn to walk in faith and follow your favor!

Don't forget to plant seeds within your heart to make you hustle with everything in you! You're going to need that to truly achieve success. Health is wealth. So, stay healthy, and the rest will follow.

 Repeat this affirmation 3 times

I can't thank the Most High enough for blessing me with the courage to face defeat.
Although it is a battle, it is already won.
Forever will I be purposefully indebted to the creator.
Thank you, Father, for loving me despite my flaws

DAY 10
I WILL GET MY LIFE ALL THE WAY TOGETHER WITHOUT APOLOGIES!

God is the cleverest of them all. You give up, and God says, "Not today." So many times, we get upset about what God is doing. But just chill, shawty. Whatever you are going through today... hang in there. God has a blessing with your name on it.

Here is a word of advice:

Don't stop, get it! Get it!

Get what you ask!
Get your life!
Get your goals!
Get your happiness!
Get out your feelings!
Get aligned with God!
Go get your blessing!

Don't stop until you're satisfied.

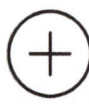

 Repeat this affirmation 3 times

This is my year of YES!
I will seek and obtain everything owed to me.
I will fight for my dreams and execute on my purpose.
I will get everything owed to me plus interest.
I will get my life!

Day 11
YOU MAY SEARCH FOR LOVE NEAR & FAR ONLY TO REALIZE THAT THE LOVE OF GOD IS IRREPLACEABLE.

God's love teaches us to forgive those who betray, love those who hate us. Also, pray for those who fail to respect you. When you love our creator, you learn to love yourself regardless of the ups and downs that imbalance the worldly mind. Sometimes our plans fail because our life's journey may be imperfect in our eyes. But when we look around... only to realize that it was God moving us through our struggles the entire time.

This is a moment for the expression of pure joy!!! Maybe it hasn't happened yet because some dreams are bigger, and we think they're too much to bear... but God!!! An imperfect dream is still the perfect dream!!! These are dream facts! Let's take our time getting to our dreams... enjoy the ride.

Repeat this affirmation 3 times

My dream is still cooking. I don't plan on quitting at all. It's my destiny to win.

DAY 12
LIFE IS FULL OF LOSSES, FAILURES, AND HARDSHIPS. THEY DON'T MAKE US QUIT.

Stop using losses as an excuse to settle the score with your ability to quit. You deserve better. Your family deserves better! Be prepared to foster your happiness every day, regardless of your dismay about life. Learn to appreciate life and all the rainy days and especially the sunny days.

Never Settle because Kings & Queens do not settle! We lead! We dream! We execute plans and visions for the most optimistic future and act on our dreams! Never waste time focusing on pleasing people. Know that as long as you and God have an understanding, everything else is irrelevant!

Like the song says, "As long as he is with me... there is no place I'd rather be." - (Rather Be by CleanBandit) Even when the storms get so bad that it looks like you may fail, stay strong.

Your story is still being written.

 Repeat this affirmation 3 times

God is writing my story. I trust the author, for His pen is flawless and miraculous.

No loss, failure or hardship is enough to make me quit

DAY 13
CREATE GOALS AND EXECUTE

    Tackle your goals and never let your foot off the pedal. Use your time wisely, and you will notice the leaps of progress towards your dreams. Don't put your goals & dreams on hold, waiting for the perfect opportunity. Those are rare and few. So, cheers to those making it happen with what you have. Focus on increasing your organization skills. Write down your goals every day.

    You don't need to fit in to make your life successful. Stop trying to follow others and create your own path. If each of us sticks to who the creator intended for us to be, there would not be many duplicates. Break out of the box... You even break the box! This world is too big and full of opportunities to help you on your journey to freedom, peace, and understanding!!! If you desire to live your dreams + you're still too comfortable... You are in the box!

 Repeat this affirmation 3 times

I am different and one in none.
My spirit, energy and favor don't fit inside a box.
I will shine and rise.

DAY 14
FOCUS ON THAT WHICH PUSHES YOU TO EXCEL TOWARDS YOUR PURPOSE & PASSION.

Eliminate the distractions that create a false sense of defeat. Aspire for goals that elevate your mind out of its comfort zone! Nothing is impossible because, with God, everything is possible! Dream Big and consistently execute your plans with strategy and precision. Carrying extra baggage into your future will only weigh you down. Eliminate toxic people, dead situations, dead food, and dead energy.

Allow your mind the opportunity to appreciate the past enough to leave it there. You haven't seen anything yet; just wait until you see why God had you wait. His surprise is worth it. God wants us to move forward and propel into our purpose with gratitude and gracefulness! Kings & Queens, now is your time to shine!!! Life is about living! Stop acting like you're dead already!

Are you ready to live yet?

Are you ready to increase your income and achieve financial freedom?

Make a checklist of all the things holding you back and plan how you will eliminate them.

Repeat this affirmation 3 times

I no longer have time for stress.
I can only devote time to things that allow me to live my best!
I will excel towards my purpose!

DAY 15
LOVE ISN'T COMPLICATED.

Love, equality, and quality must co-exist. Unfortunately, so many of us confuse love with a heap of other actions, including lust, lies, and betrayal. In my opinion, equality and quality are absolute requirements to express true love between two people. If you want to be with someone loving and kind, you should aim to exude love and kindness. If you desire someone ambitious and outgoing, your spirit must adapt to attract that. No relationship will prosper, in a healthy fashion, if two people are not equal, or if they are equal but fail to consider the quality of their attributes.

Love is simple; it can remain simple if we remember to treat others how we desire to be treated. But more importantly, if we remember to keep God in all the ways we love others (especially our opposite, our equal, our soulmate), all the complications of love will begin to vanish, just like the dew of midnight.

Find new ways to express love towards your family or significant other. Go on a date night with a spouse, take your kids on a weekend trip to bond, go on a family picnic. Make love easy.

Repeat this affirmation 3 times

Love is not complicated because God is Love.
I deserve to receive love, and I deserve to give love in return.
I love myself.
I love others.

DAY 16
MY TIME AND VIBES MATTER

In route to success, positive vibes only syndrome acts as a mental weapon to guard against any ill feelings about your goals. Sometimes we can even talk ourselves out of being elevated because of fear. But fear and doubt are the #1 killers of dreams, goals, and aspirations. Promote your mind to the next level of thinking. The new, more positive you will require next-level security and control of your thoughts. Your habits dictate your success. Make it a habit today and every day forward to monitor your vibes and control your thoughts.

Try to detox from social media, television, and music for at least 5 minutes per day for some soul mediation. Learn to listen to your inner spirit minus the distractions of daily life. Listen to your thoughts. Our subconscious mind makes up nearly 90% of the mind. The only way to use it is to turn off the conscious thoughts. Go somewhere alone, or take a brisk (non-exercising walk), and allow your mind to wonder. If any negative thoughts arise, eliminate them. After the designated time of self-meditation, feel free to write any residual positive thoughts or affirmations that come to mind in your journal.

⊕

Repeat this affirmation 3 times

My mind is my weapon.
I will treat it with respect and listen to my most inner thoughts.
Thinking positively fuels my mind with the energy it needs to reign supreme.

DAY 17
GOD BLESSED ME ABUNDANTLY!
I AM MORE THAN ENOUGH!

No matter what you have or don't have, you are royalty. Own it this very moment and never forget this. Our knowledge and ability to overcome obstacles are exceptional and elite. Many times in life, it may seem difficult to find strength during a storm, but we must learn to remain strong through adversity. Affliction affords our minds the ability to grow exponentially. After overcoming misery, something amazing transpires, we shed our fear.

We become even stronger by refusing to accept negativity or failure as an option. Even if we fail to visualize an option, sometimes we create our own solutions. Remain in a Positive Vibes Only state of mind because you are more than enough. Meditate and be still. God always has a solution if we are willing to listen actively without fear nor doubt. We are works in progress, but each day gets easier and easier.

Repeat this affirmation 3 times

I am more than enough.
Affliction will never stop me!
God blessed me abundantly!

DAY 18
CHOOSE YOUR VIBES WISELY. CHAOS CREATES WEAKNESS!

Being obedient to the creator rewards the biggest blessings of them all. Keep your head high no matter what. Deep inside your spirit lies your strength. Find it. Butterfly vibes come through just when you least expect it. That gut feeling when you're at the brink of greatness will guide you. Take that leap of faith; you know you want to!

If you're not where you want to be, why are you in a relaxed state of mind? Chilling all the time? Is peace a priority in your life or attention? What are some of the methods you use to relax? The decision may not be easy, but I promise you, it's worth it. What helps you find your purpose in life?

Our daily mood should be to write down our goals, plan, execute that plan and then get out of God's way.

Repeat this affirmation 3 times

God, I know you are working.
That's why I rise and grind every day!
God, I know you see me.
That's why I focus and hustle no matter what.
My vibes won't let me lose!
God won't allow me to fail.

DAY 19
IF A FLOWER ISN'T GROWING IT'S DYING.

You don't look like what you've been through. You're blessed. Yeah, you may have a couple of wounds and bad memories, but those have no effect on your passion and intention to win. Those many nights you spent dreaming about a way out of poverty, homelessness, and generational curses meant something. They drove you to form a plan to visualize a better life. Yes, it was hard, but you made it! God is still molding your path, but you MUST refuse to settle. This is your season; claim it.

The problem with failing is that most people see it as an automatic excuse to give up. But if you know like I know... Failure is a part of the success process. Without it, we will never grow. Failure just means that we must try again but with a new approach. Anybody successful has failed and probably very often. Failure scares me but is always the wake-up call that gets me closer to my dreams.

What is the #1 motivator that drives you to keep fighting for your goals after a setback?

Will you be intentional about your future, or will you continue leaving your day and time to chance?

 Repeat this affirmation 3 times

This is my season. I claim it.
I am going to touch so much peace, joy, and positivity this year.
My finances are covered in abundance.
My dreams keep growing and growing.
I will be intentional in this next season.

DAY 20
NUMEROUS ATTEMPTS WILL BE MADE IN THIS LIFETIME THAT WILL CHALLENGE YOUR FAITH, BUT NEVER WAVER. ⊕

This, too, shall pass. Faith is required over everything. As you approach the level of Positive Vibes Only Syndrome, you must continue detoxing everything, not benefiting your physical and spiritual growth. Eliminate things that don't bring you joy! Your mind is the most valuable asset you own. It's a terrible thing to waste. Step out on faith. Make it a habit to be your best and give yourself the time and fuel you desire to increase your joy! YOLO = You only live once. You must be prepared for your blessings, or they will pass you by. Don't be afraid to accept your calling in life no matter how much you must sacrifice. The bigger the sacrifice, the more abundant the reward.

Prepare to receive your blessings. They will be so big you may not even have room to fit them in your current house. They may be so big that you can't help but smile and let your light shine in the world. Don't be the dummy still waiting around, running from your passion. Be the King or Queen you desire to be! Don't let anyone hold you back. Keep smiling! Keep striving! Own your positive vibes and never disrespect your morals.

 Repeat this affirmation 3 times

It's my season.
I am stronger because I didn't allow my weakness to determine my destiny!
I will be positive, period!

DAY 21
ALWAYS BELIEVE THE FUTURE HAS LIMITLESS POSSIBILITIES!

Push forward! Having the Positive Vibes Only Syndrome will change your life and mindset. No longer will you engage in conversations or energies that fail to bring joy to your spirit. Be intentional about every level of your goals and purpose. Make your intentions clear and plain. The sky does not set the limit because there are no limits except wasted time. Miracles are in progress in your life. Whatever mission leads to your passion and purpose, go for it! Time waits for no man, so stop doubting yourself and waiting until tomorrow! Step out on faith to claim your ultimate success NOW.

Laziness and procrastination are two things to avoid along the journey. Wake up and dream. Find sources of inspiration daily. There are no more excuses!

What are you willing to remove from your life to gain peace of mind?

Faith over fear at ALL times and at all cost!!!

Repeat this affirmation 3 times

I'm up and chasing my goals today. I will continue chasing the intangible riches that bring pricelessness to my life! I am rich in faith. I am blessed abundantly and highly favored. I will never quit on myself regardless of my obstacles.

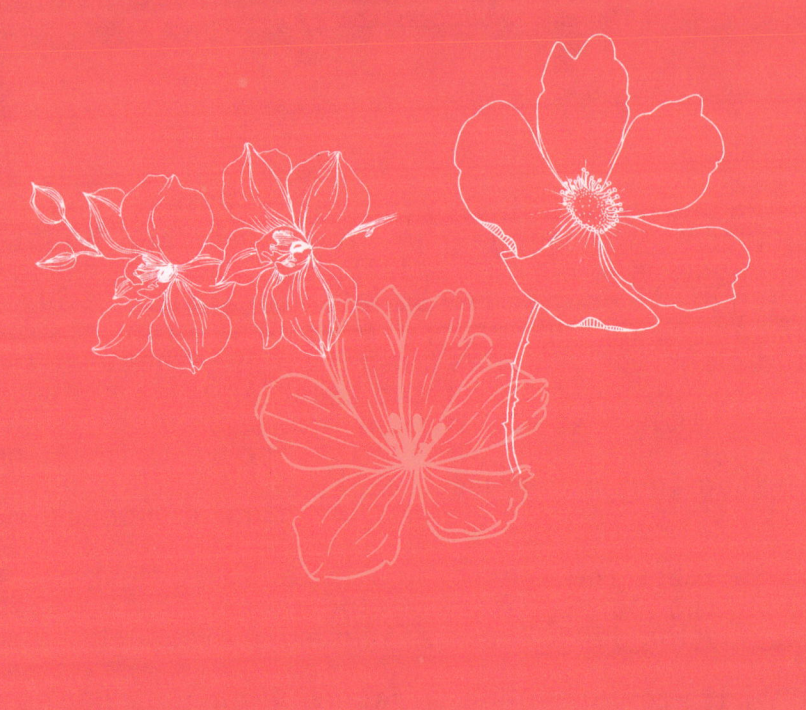

Meditation Moment

Set a timer for 5- 10 minutes.
Find a quiet place to sit alone (DO NOT DISTURB).
Close your eyes. Take slow, intentional deep breaths.
Block out all thoughts that come to your mind.
Envision being surrounded by peace and serenity.
Listen to the responses from your calmer mind.
After the timer ends, journal your thoughts.

Dr. Shon Inc.

SENDING POSITIVE VIBES ONLY! IT'S A SYNDROME!

MAINTAINING YOUR P.V.O.S. WHAT'S NEXT?

ANSWER THESE QUESTIONS:

WHAT STEP WILL YOU TAKE TODAY TO ENSURE THAT YOU PROTECT YOUR ENERGY DURING A GOOD OR BAD DAY?

WHAT IS YOUR GO-TO AFFIRMATION FOR A BAD DAY OR BAD NEWS?

WHAT IS YOUR DAILY AFFIRMATION TO SPARK YOUR GOOD VIBES ONLY?

WHAT PASSION FUELS YOUR DESIRE TO LIVE YOUR BEST LIFE?

IDEAS:

CREATE YOUR AFFIRMATION (TRY IT DOWN BELOW)

WRITE YOUR GOALS AND NEW POSITIVITY TECHNIQUES IN A DAILY JOURNAL. THIS TECHNIQUE WILL HELP TO KEEP TRACK OF YOUR MOOD AND STAY ALERT TO FIND YOUR POSITIVE AND NEGATIVE TRIGGERS.

Write Your Own Affirmation Here:

_____

_____

_____

_____

NOTES

Write Your Own Affirmation Here:

NOTES

Write Your Own Affirmation Here:

....

....

....

....

....

NOTES

Write Your Top 3 Goals Here

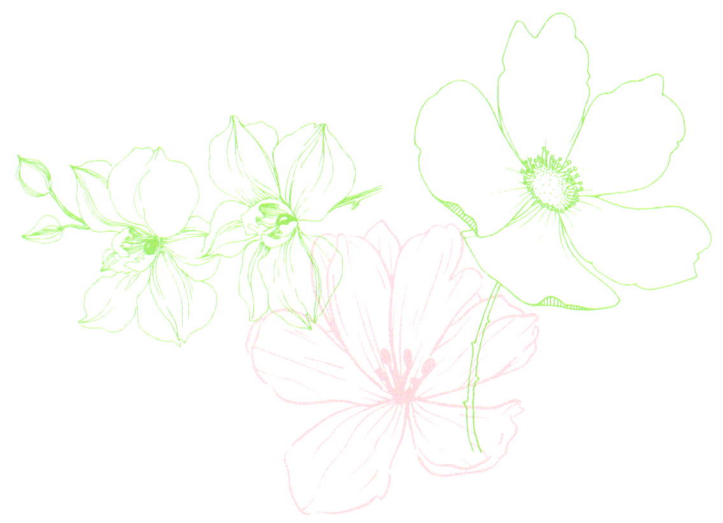

Meditation Moment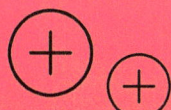

Set a timer for 5- 10 minutes.
Find a quiet place to sit alone (DO NOT DISTURB).
Close your eyes. Take slow, intentional deep breaths.
Block out all thoughts that come to your mind.
Envision being surrounded by peace and serenity.
Listen to the responses from your calmer mind.
After the timer ends, journal your thoughts.

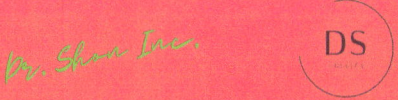

SENDING POSITIVE VIBES ONLY! IT'S A SYNDROME!

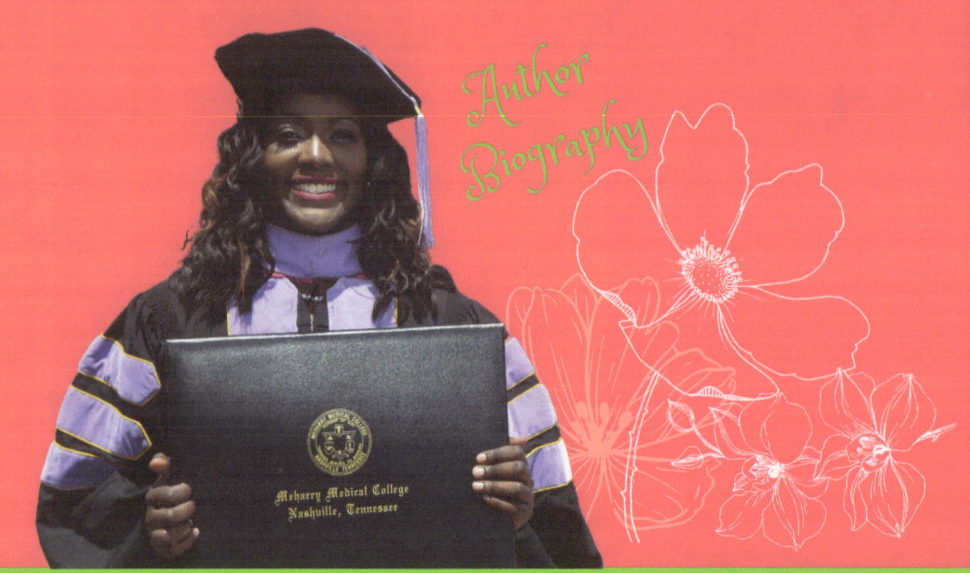

Author Biography

Shonteral Lakay Redmond, D.D.S. was born and raised in Tallahassee, Florida. She attended several grade schools due to constant custody battles between her two grandmothers after losing her mother, Doris Denise Jackson, in a fatal car accident. Shonteral was only seven years old at the time.

Despite these hurdles, she continued to defy statistics and break generational curses by enrolling into college at Florida State University. After graduating in 2009, she went on to earn a Master's Certificate in Health Sciences at the University of South Florida ('12). By the grace of God, hustle, and sacrifice, she was adorned with her Doctoral Degree in Dental Surgery from Meharry Medical College in Nashville, Tennessee, as a member of the Class of 2016.

Dr. Shon currently practices in New York as the Motivational Dentist. She also enjoys philanthropic work (The Doris Denise Jackson Foundation & DDJ DReamergency Walk), entrepreneurship, family time, and positive vibes only, of course!

Dr. Shon Inc.

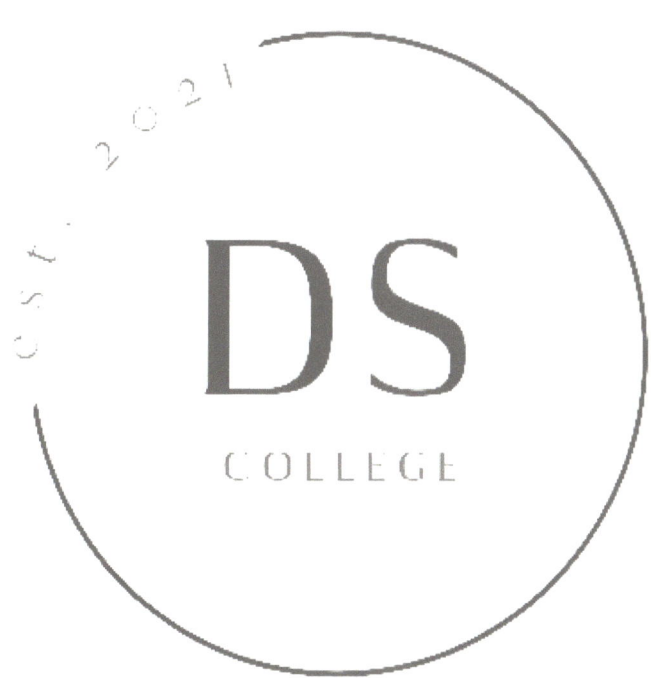

Dr. Shon Inc.

SENDING POSITIVE VIBES ONLY! IT'S A SYNDROME!

BOOKS/EBOOKS

DS COLLEGE

DORIS DENISE JACKSON FOUNDATION

DREAMERGENCY WALK

MOTIVATIONAL DENTISTRY

"MOTIVATING YOU TO TREAT YOUR TEETH LIKE ANGELS!

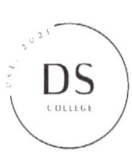

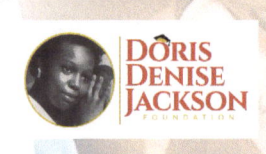

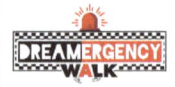

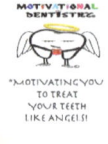

SENDING POSITIVE VIBES ONLY! IT'S A DAILY SYNDROME!

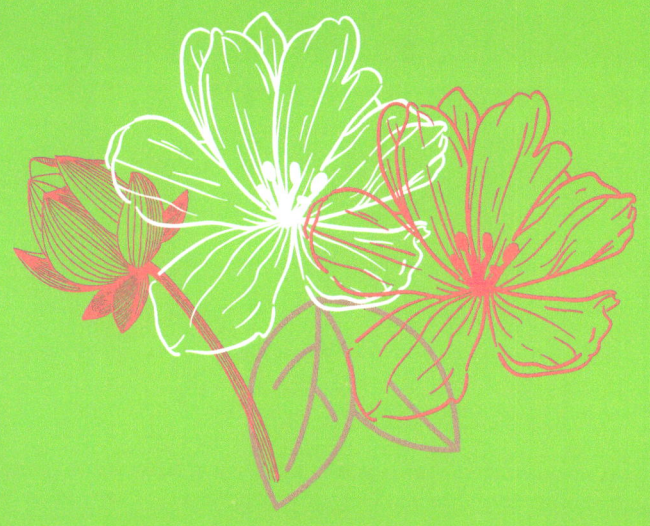

Register for the P.V.O.S Course on drshon.com

info@drshon.com

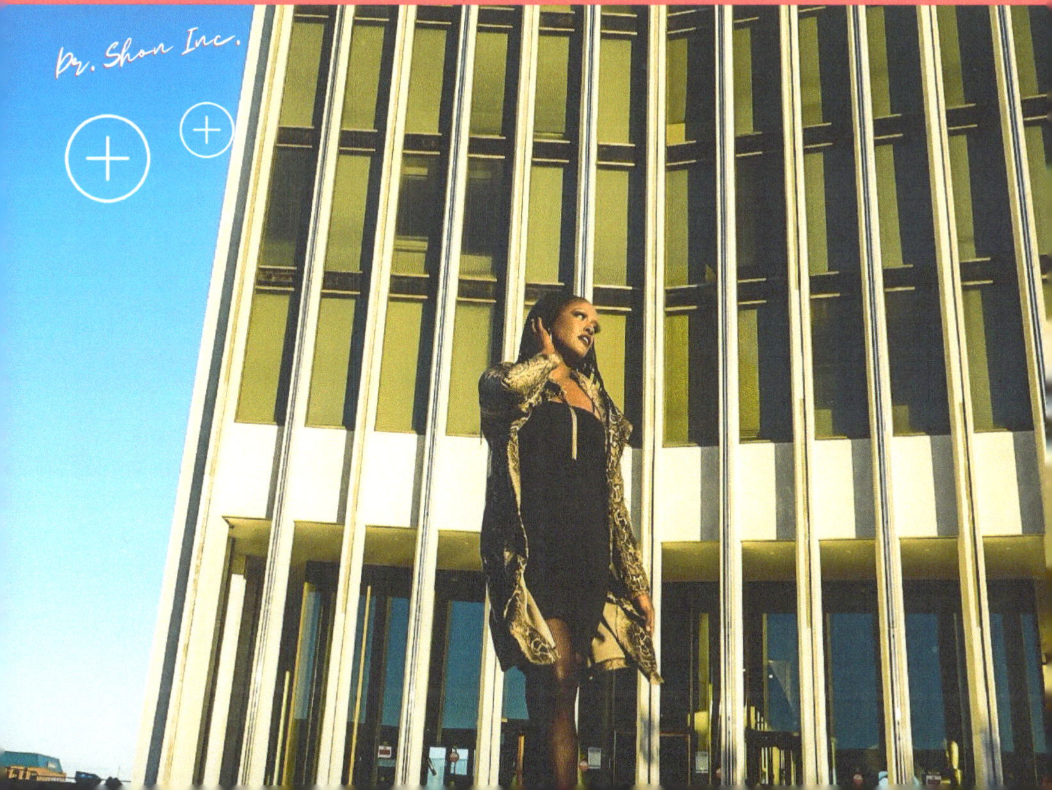

Dr. Shon Inc.

www.ingramcontent.com/pod-product-compliance
Lightning Source LLC
Chambersburg PA
CBHW040457240426
43665CB00038B/16